LISTEN TO THE WHISPERS

. . . a walk in Widowhood

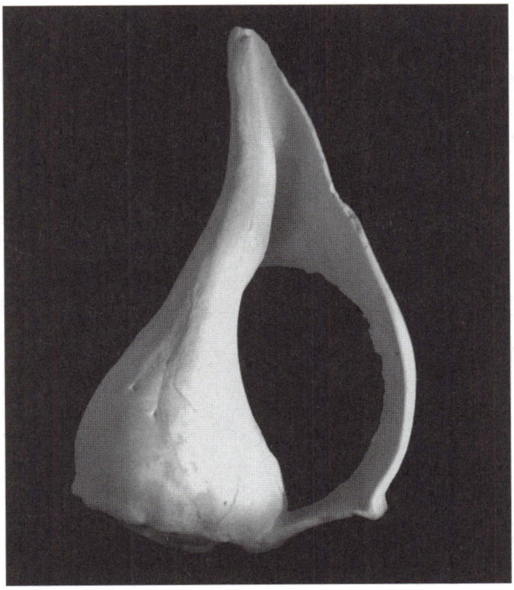

by

Elizabeth P. Lane

Listen to the Whispers

. . . a walk in Widowhood

Elizabeth P. Lane

Design & Photography: Terry M. Purdy, Cartersville, Georgia

ISBN 978-1-60585-172-3

In Loving Memory of Rudy Lane

Dedicated to Paige and Robyn
(the best daughters a Mother could ask for)

Acknowledgements …

In grateful appreciation to family: Blair, Rhodes, Alle, David, Ann Garner, Lanie, Deni, Bill, Kyle, Jarad, A.W., Carrie, Beth, Duff, Whitney, Tyson, Kris, Don, Kelly, Tyler, Terry, Carla, Allyson, Mike, Debbie, Shane, Kate, Ben, Jeremy, Hilda, Vickie (in no special order)—your calls, cards, and letters are what kept me going – I love you!

In special appreciation to friends: Patti and Ann, Bob, Dee and Allen, Tim, Pat, Hall, my Trinity family, and too many others to name, but you certainly know who you are – I thank you!

And in Special Appreciation to my **Out-of-the-Box**: Barbara and Kaye (originals), Elaine, Cheryl, Betty B., Betty C., Janet, Glenda, Ann, Reba, Jean, Brenda, Susan, Anne, and Faye – Your journeys are what it's all about!

CONTENTS

FORWARD

Your life stops right there. Just stops. And when it starts up again, it's different. It's never what it was before that moment. Never.

—— Nora Roberts (Novel - *Black Rose*)

For those of you who have not experienced this chapter in your life, this is the story no one ever tells you: the absolute loneliness, the fear of the unknown, the monumental task of building a new You, much less a new life.

For those of you who are Fellow Travelers, this is a book of Hope. I want you to know you are not alone, and I want you to know you are not crazy. You have memory lapses; you talk to your loved one; you do not have the energy to face another day, much less to deal with another legal request or even to answer the phone. It's OK.

For a long time I truly believed life does not get better after the death of your loved one, or even easier; I believed it just became different as you filled the void with life of a different concept. Through time, I have found I was wrong. With time, you adjust, and perhaps that is what makes life easier. As time passes, you become more and more thankful for the moments, weeks, months, years, you shared with your loved one.

You realize you are grateful for the shared impact you both had on each other's life. It becomes a love story of a different dimension, one that can never be taken from you. Treasure the memories, for they are what sustain you over the rough spots of the future.

Life changes in an instant.
The ordinary instant.

—— Joan Didion

You will rebuild yourself, and you will rebuild your life. You don't have a choice. Your new life will be what ***YOU*** make it. Make it the best that you can be.

Make it so in memory of your loved one. What else would they expect?

Thanks be to God, and Listen to the Whispers . . .

DEATH – THE WORST HAS HAPPENED

I had heard my sister-in-law, Debbie, a Baptist minister's wife, say many times after some happening, "It's not the worst thing that can happen." Finally, after a really deep finger cut and many stitches, I commented on the pain and near tragic experience. Yes, she voiced this thought once again. I suddenly said, Well, Debbie, what ***is*** the WORST thing that can happen?

I still remember the scene. We were in the kitchen preparing a Holiday dinner. She turned slowly and just stared at me. She then said very quietly, "Death, Beth. Death is the worst thing that can happen."

I was stunned. Of course. How could I not know? I am there.

Trust me, until you have experienced the death of your spouse, your soul mate, your child, someone really close, you do not fully comprehend or truly understand or even appreciate that statement.

You are suddenly thrown into a new life, one you did not ask for and one you did not want. You are now part of a 'different' group of people. Your friends, and sometimes your family, do not know what to do with you. You are different now, and they do not know how to deal with that difference. That's OK. You don't know how to deal with you either. Each day is a new experience, one you don't even want to face. But you do.

You don't have a choice.

This book is about this new US.

The 'ripple effect' – the way selfless acts can have an impact on more than those who are served directly, by influencing those who simply observe.

(Tyler & Day by Day)

The day before I read this, my grandson, Tyler, had given me encouragement saying if this book only helped one person, the ripple effect would create the helping of many.

Grief has no Timetable

I have always believed there was no timetable for grief. A friend said to me she had been told you don't have the right to grieve after a year. Without thinking, I replied, "Bulls…!" I realized again it was time for me to write this book. If I have learned one thing, it is DO NOT compare and DO NOT judge. Your grief is your own, no one else's. And no one has the right to tell you to move on. I have also learned that the grief process cannot and should not be hurried.

Joan Didion wrote in her book, *A Year of Magical Thinking:* "Grief turns out to be a place none of us know until we reach it." Only you know.

Because I tell you there is no timetable does not mean that you cannot move on with your life. We do – we have to. I have a friend who travels and entertains on a regular basis, but she confided in me she knew she would grieve the rest of her life. Another friend did most of her grieving while her ailing husband was alive. Her grief has been a long and strenuous path .

The evidence of what I knew I read in an article in the magazine 'O' – December 2006 – written by the news reporter, Lynn Sherr. She had spent six years knowing her husband was dying and several more years trying to find closure. Her breakthrough came in a story she was doing for 20/20 on the agony of loss. Interviewing Jimmie Holland, a pioneering psychiatrist at New York's Memorial Sloan-Kettering Cancer Center, Dr. Holland said the medical profession had been putting people into stages for years and encouraging a certain amount of time to grieve and then move on. Her words to Lynn were, "Well, wrong! You can't do this to people. Your pattern of grief is as unique as your pattern of love." She freed Lynn to mourn and to know it was not self-indulgence. It was a wonderful two page article I sent to my Out-of-the-Box group. Lynn ended saying she had finally learned to live without her husband, but not to forget him, and "to honor the memory of what was, while functioning in the world that is."

Isn't this what we all want and strive toward? The timetable is yours, and don't let anyone tell you otherwise. REMEMBER AGAIN: Do Not Judge; Do Not Compare.

Have patience with all things, but chiefly have patience with yourself.

—— Saint Francis DeSales

Rushing to Stay Busy is Normal

After the initial time, which I call The Peace Period, I went through a period of all-consuming busyness, rushing constantly to fill the hours. My daughter, Paige, had just started a new business. I volunteered to help, so I would not have to think. I only went to my own office as I needed to or had to. My husband's workshop was there also; it was too much of a reminder. On weekends I rushed to grandchildren's ballgames. I worked so hard at staying busy and on the go that my youngest daughter, Robyn, became worried about my health and well being. At that time she was a Personal Trainer for several older ladies who had been widows for years. She expressed her concern to one of her clients who only smiled and said,"It's a phase, Robyn. This too shall pass." And it did.

I still believe the key to taking steps forward is in staying busy. But I no longer have to fill every minute and rush from one thing to the next. I can sit with silence and just 'be.'

Do not fear mistakes. There are none.

—— Miles Davis

Emotions are Normal

My friend, Pat, in North Carolina, moved to Georgia at the time of her first anniversary. She had been dealing with health issues for herself and her daughter during this first year; she had put her grief on a shelf. On this first anniversary, she related experiencing all five elements of grief in one horrible day. She said she had read these were commonly shared emotions for the grief process, which she had not yet encountered.

Denial

Guilt

Anger

Grief

Acceptance

She was referring to the most commonly known elements experienced by those who lose a loved one. Please know that this in no way means you have to experience all five.

When she first related these to me, I thought I had escaped two: Guilt and Anger. I know this is true of anger, because my husband, Rudy, had such a good attitude of acceptance – how could I have less? Faith is my key. I thought GUILT was escaped until later I realized that all the first basketball games I would sit, with tears in my eyes, feeling HE should be there instead of me. In my heart I know he was there, just in another dimension.

Listen to the Whispers . . .

Do Not Judge
Do Not Compare
Do Something for Someone Else

—— epl

Grief feels Tangible

Grief feels tangible in the early stages. It engulfs us as a cloud. We walk in its haze. We feel it and taste it, as it touches us in the deepest parts of our soul. Time lifts the cloud; but, as we all know, fog can roll back over us at the most unexpected times.

Martha Whitmore Hickman wrote these words:

" I will watch for other travelers on the way who may need my help, as I need theirs."

This is why I am writing this book. I want others to hear and know that this grief and mourning is a time in which things as we knew them are suspended. What we feel and experience is 'normal' to each of us. As Joan Didion wrote in her book, *The Year of Magical Thinking*, "we are not "crazy" as in the mental and medical definition or sense. We have gone through a major shock. We are affected in all parts of our body. This means our mind as well as our heart. We do not think straight; it is hard to make decisions; our attention span is shorter. This is OK; we are not 'crazy.' We are lethargic; some days it is hard to even function. This is OK; again, we are not 'crazy.' We talk to our loved one; some of us even feel anger. It is normal; we are not crazy."

This too shall pass.

In the end, the object of what I write is not so much that people will know me and my stories so much as it is that they will know their own stories and then perhaps themselves a little better.

—— Robert Benton (author)

LIFE'S NEW CHAPTER

If you are reading this, the chances are you are in a new chapter of your life. You may have been thrown in as I was, or the approach may have been slowly occurring for a terrible and aching period of time. Regardless, you did not choose this chapter; you do not want it. The bottom line is – we have to live it. How do we get to the next chapter? Is there a next chapter? How do we become whole again?

Please let me emphasize - I do not write this to set an example. I do not write this to be a mentor. Again, I write this as a fellow traveler and, perhaps, friend. I write this to say what you are experiencing is normal; it is OK. It is OK to be confused. It is OK to hurt physically and emotionally. It is OK to cry. You are not "crazy."

You are unique. This chapter of your life is yours. The slate is clean for you, and you write the words. You LIVE the words. Sometimes the words stack, day upon day, like pancakes. Some days the words fall like blocks. And, believe it or not, some days the words are brief rays of sunshine peaking through the clouds.

In my searching for relief and understanding, I read many books. One of these described this period as a black hole that you have to walk into in order to get through. Perhaps you feel you were thrown into this darkness, and you see no light.

REMEMBER THIS: You cannot rush this chapter. You have no choice; you have to live it. Some people feel they can rush this, but it always seems to come back and haunt them at a later date.

This was not intended to be a religious book; however, I will tell you this. I could not have made this walk without my faith. I know God carried me through the 'worst.' I vividly remember experiencing the wonderful calmness that was like a protective veil engulfing me throughout the time of the funeral and continuing for a time afterwards. One of my daughters even commented on my patience with the grandchildren. I also remember vividly losing this calmness. The grandchildren had spent the night, and we were getting ready for church. I lost my cool when they weren't getting ready and were still playing. I suddenly realized the "peace" was gone. Reality had set in.

I wanted the 'peace' back, but I could not retrieve it. New steps were in front of me, and there was no direction to go but forward.

Please remember that the experiences I relate do not mean the same ones will or should occur with you. Again, REMEMBER: Your story is unique to you, and it should be. I only relate mine to stress the words again – It's OK. Hopefully, and this is definitely the intention, you will find some comfort in the words of a fellow traveler.

Woman must come of age by herself – she must find her true center alone. If one is out of touch with oneself, then one cannot touch others.

—— Anne Morrow Lindbergh

Healing – When?

Sometime in the first year after my husband's death, I attended a church dinner called Ladies' Night Out. Several widows hovered around me, in concerned love. One assured me it does get better, in time. Another one spoke up and said, "When? I still relive the night he died, over and over."

Isn't this what we all feel at times? As I have stated, I used to feel: "It doesn't get better; life becomes different as we rebuild it. And some call 'this' better." While this is true, I was also wrong. Time works curiously and slowly while we are not even aware.

Margaret Hickman Whitmore wrote:

We will not always be at this point of Altered Reality. We will, in time, incorporate our loss into our lives so that it is part of the daily background of living.

Many of you are still at a stage where you cannot imagine this part of your grief being part of your background. Trust me. It will happen.

This doesn't mean I do not still have times that my insides ache for my love and our life together. Trust me. The bursts of depression happen less frequently and are shorter in time. The love is still there, just on a different level.

REMEMBER THIS: *We must be willing to get rid of the life we've planned, so as to have the life that is waiting for us.*

—— Joseph Campbell.

This quote has been the hardest of all for me. I feel your incompleteness; I feel your aloneness.

Take my words in, and know you are not alone.

When one door closes another door opens; but we so often look so long and so regretfully upon the closed door, that we do not see the ones which open for us.

—— Alexander Graham Bell

HEALING TAKES TIME

As part of my "healing" I initiated an **Out-Of-The-Box** dinner group. I started with two, to whom I had been sending notes of encouragement. I wanted to start cooking again, even if it was once a month. Cooking had been a joy my husband and I shared, but I did not find joy in cooking for one. (Are you relating?) I decided to remodel my kitchen, cosmetically, to make it my own and perhaps add credence to my new **Out-of-the-Box** decision. My husband was a wonderful cook, and we shared many happy hours there cooking together. (Do you see the pattern?) I was searching for joy.

This has become a wonderful group of new friends. I send out invitations for a mostly monthly dinner. I follow up with recipes used that night, as well as words of encouragement. We now have 18. We did not solicit new people – they appeared. We don't have an agenda. We just have something to look forward to, with fellow travelers. We are each stepping-out-of-the-box in attending, because, number one – it's an effort and, number two – we did not know each other very well and sometimes not at all. If we feel like crying, or talking about what we are going through, it is OK; because we are fellow travelers. The Purpose is to reach out and help someone . The result is to also help ourselves.

We are each, myself included, encouraged to take a risk and step out of our comfort zone. Again, I stress not comparing. Just as we all hurt differently, we all take steps differently. What is a small risk to one person may be a hugh risk to another. What may have been quite normal in your 'other' life may now seem monumental. I encourage my out-of-the-box friends to "step out" at least once during the month. The victory is theirs. They only have to share it if they so desire. One of the ladies shared early on buying fresh flowers just for herself.

Other suggestions for Stepping-Out-Of-Your Box may be:

- Going to a restaurant alone
- Having a dinner party as a single
- Renting a video for yourself (it's amazing how little things are suddenly daunting)
- Going to the movie alone
- Buying a piece of art – just for yourself
- Having a massage – why not?
- Taking a trip alone or with acquaintances (not necessarily close friends)

- Changing the way you dress
- Changing hair style or color
- Read a book uncharacteristic for you (you might like it!)
- Listen to different music
- Volunteer
- Take art lessons

Some or all of these probably have been a normal part of your 'other' life; now they may seem huge. Set a goal for yourself – ***your*** goal – STEP OUT at least once a month too. You will be amazed at what each small victory will do for your self-esteem. Begin to care about yourself.

Healing begins with caring.

—— Bill Moyer

OK to Cry

It is acceptable and perfectly normal to cry. Martha Whitmore Hickman wrote:

No more apologies. My tears are my healing. Perhaps, too, my tears will give others permission to cry when they feel the need.

This is so true. Record it in your heart.

Grief is non-denominational. Each person is unique; therefore, their grief is as unique as yours to you.

In my readings, I found this wonderful and revealing anonymous quote:

If someone cries in front of me, I consider it a gift.

I now fully understand and feel the magnitude of that 'gift.'

As time passes and we begin to become a whole person again (and we will), we realize the hurt is still there, just as the love is still there, and will always be; but it is becoming a part of our 'inner' self. Perhaps this is what some call "getting better."

We feel we are alone in our strivings but we are not. Pain makes us reach out; and when we do, we connect and realize that others, too, have traveled along the same path. This is how we grow.

—— Alexandra Stoddard

Depression

I never thought depression was in my life, even after my husband died. I now realize it is in everyone's life. We just do not always recognize it for what it is.

When I feel lost, as I have often felt since my husband's death, I am in a stage of depression. When I am sad, it is a form of depression.

Some time after my husband's death, I was asked by my priest to attend a Lenten Study. One session would be on grief and depression. I did not feel I needed this particular segment, but he obviously saw or knew something I did not. I simply joined the group because he had called and asked me. During the particular week we touched on grief, we each had to take a private quiz, answering Yes or No to perhaps 20 questions. I was shocked to find I could answer Yes to ***all*** but the two regarding thoughts of suicide. I was depressed and did not even know it!

This was my first recognition of depression of the heart and soul. I learned a valuable lesson – depression does not have to mean you take to your bed, or that you become recluse, or that you need medication and/or counseling. Depression can take many forms and feelings. It can be, and is often, simply a deep sadness within, which can sometimes easily be hidden from others.

I am so thankful I was asked to attend that Study Group. I can, hopefully, now recognize and better respond to these deep, Normal, feelings in myself and others.

REMEMBER ALSO THIS: Do not judge others because they are not responding or acting as you feel they should or as you did. Do not judge others because they are more publicly demonstrative than you. Again, we are all unique in our grief.

When you "least" feel like it, do something for someone else.

—— Dana Reeve (Christopher Reeve's wife)

Anger – It's OK

I have read time and again that many people go through an angry stage. This is natural and part of grieving. It is not right or wrong whether or not you experience this stage.

Many of us go through constant analyzing of our feelings. I fully know and appreciate the reason I personally did not go through this stage. One of the times my husband was hospitalized with pneumonia, our priest, Tim Murphy, came to the hospital. It was early on in my husband's illness, and he had refused to share his situation unless someone specifically asked. He wanted no pity; and above all, he wanted to live a normal life. In Tim's special manner, and knowing my husband, he said, "OK, Rudy, I am just going to ask – what's wrong with you?" My husband explained he had a rare blood disease, which in layman's terms was called pre-leukemia. After he had finished explaining, Tim asked him how was his relationship with God. Rudy said, "What do you mean?" Tim wanted to know if he was angry with God because he had this disease. Rudy answered, no, he wasn't angry; why should 'he' be exempt from getting this disease; why should 'he' think he was so special as to be excluded from illness.

I have never forgotten this message. If Rudy wasn't angry, how could I be? I am truly thankful to have had this man as my husband for

19 years. It wasn't long enough, but is it ever long enough? I am simply grateful for the time we shared.

Regardless of 'my' situation, I firmly believe anger is normal. Sometimes the anger is at God. Believe me, He understands. Sometimes the anger is at our loved one for leaving us, not taking better care of themselves, or sometimes, all of the above. It doesn't have to be logical to others, or even to ourselves. It is 'our' grief, and it is OK.

The key is not to let this anger consume you. If you do, you may lose your wonderful memories. Again, the memories are what sustain us.

When you feel the anger coming on, vent it if you can (hopefully without hurting someone else). Cry if you feel like it. Then put a lid back on the can of emotions, and conjure up a good memory. Try to laugh. Keep trying this until you reach a point where you can forgive. Forgive yourself, forgive your loved one, forgive God.

If you cannot seem to get through this anger, seek professional help. Sometimes this is the only and best recourse. It's OK.

REMEMBER THIS: Keep pulling up the good memories. Try to laugh.

A day without laughter is like a day without sunshine.

—— Rudy Lane

Grief/Love

Along with the initial intensity of grief is an enormous degree of love for the one we have lost. Sometimes the two are so intertwined that, as we cling to this intensified love, we also cling to the grief. But just as the strength of true love matures in a marriage and becomes better and has flashes of intensities, we recognize we could not live at that heightened level all the time. As we recognize that the maturing of love is good, we come to also know this is what happens in the normal course of grief. This is what we want, a maturing of the grief/love. We also could not bear this intensity of grief/love for a lifetime.

The key, as I see it, is not to 'work' at 'getting rid of' the grief, for grief needs and demands its own time. Nor should we try to hold on to this intensity of the love. Love does not leave us. It matures with us, as it should.

REMEMBER THIS: Treasure the memories – keeping the good and discarding the not so good.

Bereavement of married love is but one of its regular phases – like the honeymoon. What we want is to live our marriage well and faithfully through that phase (bereavement), too.

—— C.S. Lewis – *A Grief Observed*

Listening to the Whispers

We Listen to the Whispers, because we want to believe our loved one is still there. In this new realm of awareness, we become more attuned; because we don't want to lose this bond.

I had always been afraid of death. I am no longer. I truly know my loved one is there and will be when my time comes. It was hard for me to "let go" of needing his presence. He finally came to me through a friend in a vision and said, "I am home." I experienced a great sadness and cried. I realized I was crying for myself. I had 'hung on' too long. He knew this before I did. He knew before I did that I would be OK and that it was time. This experience does not happen to everyone. But I sincerely believe it happened for me. He knew how much I still needed him, and he was there as long as he could be. Again, this does not happen to everyone.

REMEMBER: Do not compare.

I wonder. If, as I can't help suspecting, the dead also feel the pains of separation (this may be part of their purgatorial sufferings), then for both lovers, bereavement is a universal and integral part of our experience of love.

—— C.S. Lewis

THE QUESTION – HOW ARE YOU?

THE question seems to always be there. Family and friends are concerned, and they ask – How are you? Your answer is always the same – I'm fine; I'm OK; good days and bad days – routine question; routine answers.

My husband used to say when people ask how are you or how is your day, they did not expect an answer. He sometimes would play a game and say with a smile (the important part) - terrible, just lost my dog, etc. etc. The person would not even hear the answer; they just saw the smile and keep going.

Then someone "really" looks into your eyes and asks softly, " How ARE you?"

Sometimes you burst into tears. It is so hard to be honest, and it is so hard to really say, "I don't know. It's all new; one step at a time." It's the same world to everyone else. WE are the ones who are different. WE are the ones building a new life. WE are the ones with tender feelings. Our friends and family have gone back to their lives, as they should. WE are the ones looking at everything through new eyes and feeling our way across our scarred battlefield of a life. For it IS a battle to get up every morning and face the world alone when only 'yesterday' we were so happy.

So how do you answer those who really do care and honestly want to know? With simple honesty and a quiet resolve – I may not always know, but I'm working on it.

Sorrow is not a state, but a process.

—— C.S. Lewis

READING/WRITING

As is the case with many, several people gave me books after my husband died. Although I eventually read them all, the one which helped the most was *Healing After Loss*, by Martha Whitmore Hickman. It was more like a Day-by-Day, short and within my limited attention span at that time. Although I have kept my original, given by my good friend, Adrienne Ford, who had lost a son, I have purchased many copies for new widows. It speaks.

You must decide what is best for you. Reading may be your source of help or writing in a journal, or both. There is no right or wrong.

I had been told that writing in a journal was helpful. I am a 'tight' person who does not share easily. In the beginning I could not 'share' on paper, even with myself. I have another friend, who 'writes' to her deceased spouse every night. You must do what helps you.

As time passed, and I had read so few books which really helped me, I began to see that "I" might be a helper to others. I wrote first on March 21, 2004, three days after what would have been my husband's birthday. It had been one year and six months. It is now five years later. It has helped me to express my feelings. If you feel so led, perhaps you will be able to start sooner than I. No one has to read what you write. At the appropriate time, you can burn or discard the pages.

The choice is always yours.

As Martha Whitmore Hickman said, “It may help you sort things out, and you will be free to move on into the next moments of your life.”

I have taken her words to heart. (I have read her book three complete times and highlighted areas more than this.) Perhaps after writing this book, not only may it help someone else, perhaps I will better be able to move on to the next chapter of my life.

Our inner condition, rather than our outer circumstances, is what truly defines us.

—— Roger Housden

Happiness ???

C.S. Lewis wrote: N*o one ever told me about the laziness of grief, the loathing of even the slightest effort; feeling – what does it even matter now? (writing, reading, even shaving). And: Grief feels like fear and, more strictly, suspense – waiting, provisional – life doesn't seem worth starting anything. Up until this time I had too little time; now there is nothing but time – empty.* (paraphrased)

Apathy is the norm. What is happiness, but a lost feeling.

Happiness is no longer what it once was. Regardless, we still have the ability to choose happiness, perhaps not in the beginning, but at some point. It is up to each of us to bring light into our own lives again.

If you need, reread what I have just said, again and again if need be. You may be saying – You don't understand; this is impossible.

Believe me. I understand. My husband was my best friend, and he was quite simply my sun. He was my crucial light for laughter and happiness. I do know where you are.

As we try to do even simple things, they simply just are not as much fun. I know. But we have to keep trying and cheering each other on. That's right. We now have a responsibility to others who have experienced the 'worst' as we have. We are in a sisterhood/brotherhood all our own and certainly not our choosing. My way, as yours, is tentative, but yielding light, none the less, through memories, warmth of home, family, and friends, old and new.

REMEMBER THIS: "It's OK" is giving yourself permission to experience grief your way. Well meaning friends and family tell you 'they are in a better place' and 'you wouldn't want them to suffer' and 'you are being selfish' or, even worse, perhaps they avoid you altogether. Try not to take offense. They have never been in the place you are. Remember you were once in their shoes. You did not know what to say then either.

Try to take pleasure in the small things. I invite you to try, by Stepping Out-of-Your-Box. As Mick Jaggar sings,

You can't always get what you want;
But if you try sometime,
You just might find,
You get what you need.

Even, and perhaps especially, at moments of great sadness, we need to laugh.

—— *Zen Paths to Laughter*

Self Image

In this vulnerable new chapter of our lives, some of us may realize we don't like ourselves right now. Of course we don't. We've lost one half of our person. We feel deformed. But it is really our life we don't like. We want the old one back. We are insecure, as we search for our new self.

I know one woman who redid her whole house. Her daughter said – I don't know why she's doing this. I 'now' know. It was part of searching for her new identity. Some people move, even to a new town. It may appear to others to be running away. It is really part of the search.

For me, it has been my hair. I know this appears silly, but it has been very real to me. (Reminder: if you have a bad hair day, you have a bad start on your day. We all know that.) For me, my illogical part of the brain kicked into gear big time about my hair. Logically, I realize my husband was no longer here to tell me I was beautiful (of course, I'm not beautiful, but in his eyes, I was). Therefore, suddenly my hair became super important. I kept trying new styles and shades. Finally one of my daughters suggested I try someone in another town who appraised you and did it his way. It's getting better.

Thanks be to God for daughters. They have helped me with this illogical problem. They now are my re-enforcers. Of course, it is not the same; but it helps bring in the reality. They have assumed this special role which has extended into my wardrobe. All my life I have favored blacks and browns. They have brought color into my clothes. I have accepted this 'help', with mostly good nature. I keep reminding myself, it is part of my Stepping Out-Of-My Box, this new me.

They are also my strongest supporters. They are there to help me with the self-image inside as well as out. Our fragile selves need support from family and friends.

Paige: You have to find that place within where you are comfortable. (I'm still working on this.)

Robyn: If you question yourself, you damage the memories you have. (So True)

"Some things happen to us from which we never recover, and they disrupt the normalcy of our lives. We must forget 'the old standard' and accept a "new normal."

—— Don Piper

Low Energy

Low energy is normal. Sometimes it is so bad, we see a doctor to find out if something is physically wrong. I went through two and a half years with first no energy and then very low energy, with no real purpose or direction. In reflecting on this late one night with my brother, Terry, he gave me this insight:

"Beth, you and Rudy had such strong energy 'together.' With his death, you lost half of that energy. It takes time to rebuild it."

We all need to be reminded that we are human. My brother was right. This is part of making the new me.

Margaret Whitmore Hickman wrote:

I will live through these days the best I can; trusting that in time my spontaneity and energy will return.

Grief is a very private existence. We grow up hearing and saying: *Blessed are Those Who Mourn.* Of course, it is different when it happens to oneself. REMEMBER THIS: What you see on the exterior may not be what is on the inside. This is part of the Do Not Compare; Do Not Judge.

Sometimes the "best I can" is just to endure.

—— Don Piper

Melancholy

I first read of melancholy in relation to what I was experiencing in Martha Whitmore Hickman's *Healing After Loss*, 'a kind of low-key sadness.' I thought to myself: Melancholy — yes — perfect word, perfect word. Isn't this what fills our total self after the intense grief begins to slowly drift away? Faced with stark white reality, our life goes into the foggy gray zone of melancholy. And, as with fog, this feeling of sadness is sometimes extremely dense and sometimes patchy and occasionally lifts enough for rays of sunshine to peak through. Melancholy is the perfect word for this chapter of our lives. It is a blanket engulfing us in lethargy and depression during the times of dense fog and simple sadness, during the patches of fog.

We have to work on walking, with baby steps, hands outstretched, finding our way out. Some days, or parts of days, are more successful than others. Staying busy; getting a 'jobette,' as my friend Charlotte once said; volunteering; doing something for someone else helps. WE have to make it happen, the pulling ourselves out of the fog.

By the same token, if you simply cannot make it through this fog of melancholy alone, by all means, seek professional help, and quickly. REMEMBER THIS: There are certain times in our lives when we all need help. It's OK. This is not a bad thing. What would be tragic would be not getting the help needed so we can move on to the next chapter.

You have to learn to 'let' people help you. It is their way of showing their love and concern. It is their gift.

—— epl

Empty Future

Lisa Gardner used this poignant quote in her novel *Gone*:

It was not the past that broke you. It was the empty future, the endless string of days filled with none of the people who mattered most.

Once you've been in this empty void, you know and feel the gray confusion of this time. And it is a color – gray. We each have to work our own way out of this cold, damp, and dismal place. We have to learn to fill this 'empty future' day by day. But we each have to do it our own way.

What works for me (most of the time) is not to dwell on the vast void of the future and to keep busy in the present, no longer at a frantic pace, but a calm, steady busy.

Nora Roberts said in her novel, *Divided in Death: "Life is never as long as you want it to be."*

We now all know and live the stark truth of that statement.

I wish I could give you a magic answer. I wish I could say – this amount of time and it will be over. I am only a fellow traveler. I do not and cannot write this to tell you what to do or not to do. I am simply reaching out to you to say – what you are experiencing is normal; you are not crazy.

This is your time.

REMEMBER THIS:

No one can go through this for you.

Be kind to yourself.

Forgive yourself for not being the perfect wife or mother. (no one is)

Give yourself permission to grieve and mourn for as long as YOU need.

We now tend to equate happenings in our life in terms of 'before' and 'after.' This is natural. After all, we are no longer the same person we were 'before.' Our future will be what we make it.

Jerry Sittser in *A Grace Disguised* wrote:

It is not, therefore, the 'experience' of loss that becomes the defining moment of our lives . . . it is how we 'respond' to loss that matters. That response will largely determine the quality, the direction, and the impact of our lives.

I'm still working on this one.

When infinite longing comes, take a walk, write a poem, call a friend.

—— Perry E. Gresham - *With Wings As Eagles*

The Color of Grief

At a time of grief, you do not want to 'think,' and, yet, all you do is think. You relive, over and over, the actual period of dying, rethinking all possibilities, logical and illogical.

For me, the color of grief is gray. When I think about this, I realize my brother, Terry, told me I was going through a "gray" period in my life; because, as an avid collector of art, I have suddenly been drawn to, rearranged for, and added to my collection – grays, browns, and blacks. I looked around me and suddenly see this is true. I have added black and white photos, framed and matted in grays and blacks, to my walls. Two central pictures purchased in memory of my husband (a ritual started with my parents) are in dark, somber hues. One now hangs above my fireplace. It has replaced three vivid paintings of English countryside framed in white. The second one is beside my bed – also total grays. It is the first and last vision I see each day. But I find this soothing. I have added a wall of old etchings, pens and inks, dark watercolors, above my bed – a European look, but in soothing dark tones. As I would normally do, I purchased a piece of art on a trip to Charleston with friends. It spoke to me from a large park of art – grays and browns and blacks – but now with a touch of blue. Perhaps my brother is truly insightful. My Gray Period may be inspired by my grief. But, never the less, it comforts me. And, it may be as a mist of warming fog, but it is ME for now.

Once again, my point is – this is YOUR time. You are the one traveling through the 'black hole.'

Be kind to yourself. There is no easy way through grief, no way to speed up the process. You just have to live it.

It's a small fraternity, and none of us joined by choice.

—— epl

The 'Now' Person

We are no longer a 'we.' How do we discover who we are now? I wish there was an easy answer. Do this; do that; follow this plan and it will work out. It just does not happen that way. Just as we are all unique, we all must walk our own path through the maze of grief and beyond, with trials and errors. It's OK. No one is perfect.

How do we ease this pain of loss as we are trying to find our way in this new world? We don't. It's real. I do know it is a constant search. I do know I have a lot of questions I did not have before, questions about life's purpose, life hereafter, where the soul of the loved one physically is – with us unseen ? – where is heaven really, and on and on. I also know I would not have been able to bear any of this without God's help. Even though I have questions, I do not question the existence of God. I 'know' He has carried me when I could not walk.

Sometimes you need to voice how you feel with family or friends. They love you, but they cannot read your mind. They also may not be as patient as you would like or expect. You have to lead the way for them to help or listen. Just say – I need to talk about what's going on with me.

Each of us is "coming of age" in this new chapter. We have to do it by ourselves. We alone must find our true center. One has to come to terms with oneself, not only in a new stage of life, but in a new role – living for one's self and no longer a 'we.'

Grief: The raindrops of sadness; the tears of the soul.

—— epl

Lack of Self-Confidence

Just as we suddenly feel we have lost our identity and, with it, our self-confidence, we are very vulnerable and fragile. Our feelings are raw. We no longer feel confident doing things we have always done. We feel on display, the object of talk or pity. We are suddenly self-conscious.

How do we regain that control of our lives; how do we regain that self-confidence we always took for granted? Again, there is no easy answer. We have to work on it. One of the ways is stepping out of our box and doing things we don't really want to or have the energy to. We do it by helping someone else, even anonymously. Each time we do, we can be proud of ourselves. We can even 'reward' ourselves.

Alexandra Stoddard wrote: *Trust our inner consciousness. Self-awareness increases our self-confidence.*

Part of this regaining of self-confidence is, naturally, finding out – who am I now? We walk a path all our own to redefine or even reinvent this person who is ME.

Oprah wrote:

What is your purpose, what is your calling? What I know for sure is, if you ask the question, the answer will come. You have to be willing to listen for the answer. You have to get still enough to learn it and hear it and pay attention, to be fully conscious enough to see not just with your eyes but through them to the truth of who you are and what you can be.

A new friend of mine who has been a widow for some years, suggested that I think about things I might have always wanted to do but had been placed aside because it did not interest my spouse or because I had been mother and caretaker of family life. For some of us, it is a novel idea to suddenly put our wants and desires first. This is part of the healing.

Martha Whitmore Hickman wrote that coming into this personal wakefulness through grief is like giving birth with difficulty. She further encourages attention to our own needs, our state of mind through reading, rest, a willingness to be vulnerable again, counseling if needed, prayer and/or meditation, and even participation in a healing community. She adds: What we can be sure of is that we will be different.

C.S. Lewis wrote about feeling dazed, almost as if having a concussion. He expounded further by saying his life felt like it was in suspense, with thoughts, feelings, and actions that had once been directed toward the loved one and now the target is gone.

We can all choose adjectives that described that initial time, or even now. One of mine would be automatic pilot. But, at some point, we have to take the instruments off automatic. Coming back into the real world increases the pain and awareness, but it is the only way to heal and even grow. But I cannot stress strongly enough, it must be in your own time, not someone else's.

This is YOUR grief; only you know when to take the next step.

"I don't know how to exist in a world where my Dad isn't."

—— The Character 'George' in *Grey's Anatomy*

Reaching Out is Hard

Taking that step to reach out when you need to talk is monumental. A new friend who was a widow of two and a half months called to ask me to go to dinner. She probably did not know how big a step this was. I did. Even though we had talked and visited and communicated in cards, I knew in my heart what courage it took for her to call and ask me to meet her for dinner. She was at a point of intense emotions of grief and anger. However, she was one of the fortunate ones who realized she needed help and reached out. She reached out to her doctor for her depression, and she reached out to a grief counselor. I felt honored she had also reach out to me. This was good.

This is a new role for all of us. Believe me, at some point you will be in a position or will be asked to help someone else. You will do it without thinking, and it will help you. It appears that God brings people into our lives who need us, giving us the opportunity to touch their lives as someone else has touched ours.

One of the deep secrets of life is that all that is really worth doing is what we do for others.

—— Lewis Caroll

THE 'W' WORD

Especially in the beginning, we all despise the 'W' word. We still feel we are a wife, and we don't want that to change, even though it has. But, as time eases the intensity of grief, it also eases the intensity of feeling of the 'W' word. A widow is not something we want to be, and it is not something we would have chosen. It has been thrust upon you, and we are not prepared. For a long time we still feel married, so how can we accept being a Widow? I can only tell you Time and Grace eases us through this period.

I have learned to cope with the "W' word. I no longer feel it is a large black capital letter, forged on my body for all to see, as in the story of the *Scarlett Letter*. I try to remember it is an honored position in the eyes of God, honored 'W's'– Widow as well as Wife.

You just need to get past this . . . Stop going over the way things used to be. Discover what I have now and build on it.

—— Don Piper

FEAR

I see and hear fears in each of us. Fear is one of the demons we fight – fear of the unknown, fear of being alone, fear of being taken advantage of, fear of finances, fear of fear itself, and on and on.

A Day by Day author wrote: *Years ago a wise counselor spoke of a frightened little boy who walked by my side warning me of every possible pitfall and danger, making me anxious and fretful. Rather than kick or escape or deny him, she suggested my task was to take him by the hand, listen to his warnings, and tell him that together we are going to make it.*

And we are. REMEMBER THIS: We ALL have our fears. Although they are unique unto our person and situation, they are also so similar because of our circumstances.

Fears are not always of our circumstances either. Sometimes it is fear of not remembering our loved one as we did or fear of losing mental contact with our lost one. Martha Whitmore Hickman wrote: "*Sometimes we are unconsciously fearful that if we begin to move away from our grief, we will lose what contact we have with the one we miss so much.*" But maybe it is like letting go of one's children when they are ready to move off on their own. Perhaps the relinquishing of our most intense grief makes a space into which a new relationship with the loved one can move.

It is hard to face our fears, and night time is the worst. But, seemingly as a miracle, with the dawning of day, comes a better understanding and courage to face the day. However, if this is not the case with you, you may need to seek professional help if fears become overwhelming.

This is nothing to be ashamed of. It is OK.

This is an important quote for me and one I have shared with many, given to me by my niece (and adopted grandchild), Allyson:

> We cannot change the past,
> But we can ruin the present
> By worrying about the future.

You gain strength, courage and confidence by every experience in which you really stop to look fear in the face . . . You must do the thing which you think you cannot do.

—— Eleanor Roosevelt

I Loved My Life

A friend once said to me, "I loved my life. I didn't want it to end." It truly touched me, because I felt the same. This is not true for everyone. This is OK too.

My husband's sister had a very domineering husband, but she still missed his presence when he was gone. After his death, she blossomed into a new person who discovered quilting and art and developed new friends. Another friend's husband was sick for ten years, slowly ebbing away at quality of life. She experienced her major grief while he was alive. Both of these women are amazing examples to others. REMEMBER THIS: We are all different. We all experience our own grief differently.

I once wrote to my husband's daughters that I realized with a sense of wonder and love and awe that I had lived a Christmas life with their father. To me this was the most beautiful analogy I could give them of their father, because Christmas has always been my favorite time of year.

I certainly did not mean this in the gift-giving manner. I meant it in the true spirit of Christmas, a life of special love and inspiring awe and gratefulness, and, most importantly, growth together in spirituality. Our priest at the time, Tim Murphy, once said in his final sermon, expressing his gratitude for the honor of burying our loved ones and, as he recounted the names of each of our loved ones buried: *Rudy Lane, soul mate of Beth Lane, for eternity*. What a compliment!

Regardless of your situation, I emphasis once again: Do NOT Compare; Do NOT Judge.

Christmas: The bell still rings for all who truly believe.

—— Polar Express

Attention Span

In the early period of our grief, we experience many things, including disorientation, loss of memory, lack of attention span, etc. This is NORMAL!

An avid reader, I went through three months (others have told me longer for them) after my husband died that I could not read. I found I just could not concentrate for any length of time. I kept thinking I "should" find solice in reading, even an escapism, but it would not come. This is perhaps the reason I found *Healing After Loss* so welcoming. It had extremely short and manageable day- by -day readings.

I wanted to read. I wanted the comfort of reading. (This was one of the pleasures my husband and I shared.) I also wanted the escapism it would bring. I could not force it. What I did not realize at the time was 'I' was not the same person and would never be again. I was beginning the path of a new identity. This not being able to concentrate was part of the whirling process of uncertainty of this new chapter.

I truly missed this simple pleasure also. Of all the things I could no longer experience, I felt I could and must retrieve this one. I thought perhaps if I read something I would not normally have read, it might change the tide. I chose *My Losing Season* by Pat Conroy. Although I had read all but one of his books, this one I would not have chosen. It was a true story of one year in his life at the Citadel and his basketball season. It was a book for Rudy, not for me. I pressed on and made it. The book was so good that I purchased several for Christmas presents, for our best friend, Allen Cooke, and two of the grandsons, A.W. Hamilton and Tyler Lowros. Some time later I encouraged two granddaughters to read it, Whitney Jeffers and Carrie Hamilton. Another grandson read it on his own, Jarad Hamilton. It became a book for all of us. We could see Rudy (PaPa) in the book!

The key is persevering. In Joan Didion's book, *The Year of Magical Thinking*, she thought she was going crazy. She brilliantly describes the illogical thinking that occurs during this time. She vividly describes illogical decisions made (not giving away all his clothes – he might need them; not giving away his shoes – he might need them) These were non-sensical thoughts, but ones I understood. My logical side said my husband would have chastised me, saying someone else could benefit from his clothes. My illogical side knew "I" needed them more at the time; this would be fully admitting he was never coming back. Life becomes persevering. We don't have a choice. Most of our 'crazy' thoughts we can't even admit to others at the time. 'We' even question ourselves at times. This is why I stress – you are NOT crazy. This too shall pass.

My friend, Charlotte, once said, “There is a three inch hole in my head where my brain used to be. The wind whips through and takes my memory with it.” So aptly put.

Grief is a pain so great that it is almost a physical presence inside you.

—— Caroline Myss
Invisible Acts of Power

Helping Others

After we have been 'pushed' into this new chapter of our life, we suddenly realize how little we have helped others in similar circumstances before now. Although we may chastise (to no avail, I might add) ourselves, over time we realize we could not have acted any differently; because we had not experienced it first hand.

The world takes on a different look in this new chapter. We suddenly realize how very unimportant most things are. We become an 'expert' on telling others to love more, hug more, and spend more quality time with your children and spouses. Will it work? Who knows. Only those who have experienced the 'worst' can truly see the small details of ordinary happiness.

How many times in the past have we said, Call me if there is anything I can do or help you with.

"Now" we know that call will just will ***not*** take place. We just do not have the energy to call; we want to be a hermit. "Now" we know WE are the ones who have to take the initiative. "Now" WE know WE are the ones who have to take charge and make things happen for the "W."

I was fortunate in having two close friends who pushed and pulled me out of the house and made me do things and go places. Although my daughters were extremely sensitive and included me in everything, as did their spouses, I did not want to take over their lives. I did not want to become a burden to them. In trying to take charge of my life again, I joined an EFM class at church. The goal was to make myself get out of the house at night. I achieved my goal and felt a victory after a year of Monday nights. I truly enjoyed the people; the Mentor was great, but my goal had been different from theirs.

Linda Feinberg wrote in *I'm Grieving As Fast As I Can*, "It has been said that the worst symptom of grief is that you can't see any light at the end of the tunnel." YOU can't see the light, but I am here to reassure you, there ***is*** light.

You have to find your own way in this New Chapter. I cannot stress strongly enough a ***key*** to your development is helping others, often anonymously. You will find you are changed in the process. Remember the quote from Dana Reeves, do it when you least feel like it. REMEMBER THIS: Be kind to yourself; be patient with yourself.

Give because you want to touch someone.

——Alexandra Stoddard

Permission

Sometimes we are forced in life to drop our role we present to the world. Death is one of those times. In this vulnerable state, we are freer to receive the warmth and kindness of others. This is also a gift to our friends and family. Allowing them to help you, in any way, allows them to feel needed and express their love and concern.

We must give ourselves permission to be this vulnerable. It's OK to cry at inopportune times. It's OK to eat tomato soup for breakfast, as one friend said. It's OK to eat apples and cheese with wine for dinner (I survived for two and a half years on mostly this.). It's OK to say – NO – if you really don't feel like doing or going. It's OK to feel sorry for yourself (in the beginning). It's OK to not want to get out of bed (in the beginning – but do it anyway – it's the small steps that matter). It's OK to be depressed, but remember, you're the only one who can pull yourself out of depression.

Again, be kind to yourself. And again, don't compare how you are feeling or acting with anyone else. Remember, you don't know what's going on in someone else's head or behind their closed door.

The first year, almost without realizing it, we have a goal . . . ***if*** we can just get through that first year of 'firsts' and 'anniversaries' and special occasions. And then it's there. There is a sense of relief in knowing we have passed this first years of "firsts." Another friend shared with me after her first year anniversary: If I can get through this first year, I can do anything!

Please remember the "first year" is only a gauge. Many people experience much of what others go through after death during life, an ongoing battle during illness. This is also the reason I say – Do NOT Compare. Linda Feinberg said, "I don't even know what's normal anymore." This is also true for those who experience the slow death of quality of life during the living.

Know that you are your unique person and give yourself permission to react and act accordingly.

We must learn to become comfortable in our new chapter, our new environment of one.

—— epl

This is Not Me

Many of the experiences or feelings I have talked about may not have happened to you. It's OK. There is no right or wrong way to feel; no timetable for grief.

A friend of mine in another state was besieged with health problems of her own, as well as family, after her husband died. It was not until a year later, on the first anniversary of his death, that she began to grieve. Unfortunately, her 'support group' had moved on with their lives. She was intelligent enough to realize what was happening, but she had no one to turn to. She had moved to another city and was beginning a new life without the one she loved most.

If you have had none of these feelings, you are fortunate. Do NOT think there is something wrong with you. Perhaps you have had all and more. In either case, REMEMBER THIS: you are not crazy!

I began this book to help others to know they are not alone in their feelings and actions and that they are not crazy as they experience the roller coaster emotions of grief. Many times over the time period I have written, I have felt this was all, and then along would come another passage. Sometimes another book recommended to me would prompt another passage. I don't feel these were accidents.

An out-of-print book was recommended to me by a young male

widower, who had happily remarried after several years. I have mentioned a couple of quotes from the book – Linda Feinberg's *I'm Grieving As Fast As I Can*. The title became his response when he was enundated with casseroles and advised to find a mother for his four children. A specialist in grief and loss therapy, Ms. Feinberg encourages my thought process:

Consider yourself lucky if you don't have some or many of these symptoms. Don't worry about the ones you do have. You are not going crazy. You are in grief.

I have written this book for myself, as much as for you. I am reaching out to those who need to be reassured, but I am also reassuring myself. I'm OK and each day I get better. I cannot speak to you as an expert or a professional on grief; I cannot even speak to you on women's grief. I can only speak to you of my grief and my path. Perhaps it will speak to your soul. If I can help one of you, then my sharing was as it should be. This is part of the new beginning, the New Chapter.

Time removes all things but love and truth.

—— Hall Whitworth

Second Chance at Life

In one of his last sermons at my home church, my priest, Tim Murphy, told a story of a woman in her nineties walking on the beach. She came across a man throwing star fish back into the ocean. She stopped walking and, in natural curiosity, asked the man if he was a collector. He replied, no, I'm giving them a second chance at life.

That is what we are being given. As we try to figure out who we are in this new and unwanted life, isn't this what God is giving us – a second chance? We've made it through the 'worst' (with His help). Now it's time for a new chapter, granted, unasked for and unwanted; but we're in it, no less. It is up to us to make the best of our second chance and, hopefully, to help someone else along the way.

You may be at a stage where this seems too daunting. That's OK. I think this is what friends and family do not fully realize, the utter scope of this immense loss is not just a person loved and now gone. To the spouse left behind, a part of their being has ended also. The loss is not only a physical loss, but also a loss of a relationship of togetherness, a loss of expectations of a future, and, as my brother Terry so aptly put it, a loss of the sheer energy of intertwined souls. Until one has experienced the stark uniqueness unto yourself, one cannot, and should not, fully understand the extent of the loss of your best friend, your lover, the father (step-father) to your children, your mentor, your confidant, your soul mate. The list seems bottomless and so void.

Rebuilding a new you, or even thinking about a second chance on life, does seem intimidating. We drift for a while, as the wind blows, taking one day at a time. At some point the wind becomes a cool breeze and the filtered light becomes gentle rays of sunshine. We suddenly realize --- we want to live!

What a tragedy it would be not to grab that thought and take those faltering steps into the sunshine. My home and heart are full of wonderful memories I do not want to lose or give up. The goal is to build on those, as a mentor would expect you to, as a loved one would want you to..

REMEMBER THIS: The rawness and intensity does lessen. It has to or we would not survive. It will be up to each of us to make the most of this Second Chance.

My home . . . It had given me quiet, steady, demanding and undemanding seasons of pleasure. I took care of my home, then my home took care of me. Houses are patient with grief.

—— Dominique Browning - *Around the House and In The Garden*

Others Are Grieving Too

Others really are grieving too. During the funeral time we all seem to reach out to each other. It is after we are alone that we feel we are the only ones in this isolated place. Later we realize others are and were grieving, just on a different level. We are all unique, and we all had a special and different relationship with the one who is now gone.

We must remember that friends grieve, just like family. And just like family, they don't know how to react to your grief, as they also try to deal with theirs. The difference is they, just like family, go back to their lives. They can compartmentalize or even 'disappear' their grief.

We also find that a good many of our friends disappear, not necessarily because they consciously want to, but because they simply do not know what to say or do. And YOU do not know how to help them help you, because ***you*** don't know how to help yourself either. The gray fog has rolled in, and it's heavy. It engulfs you, and you can't see through it.

Some close friends, some old and some new, are persistent. They become buoys, just like family. Much later you realize they were hurting too; but it's hard, if not impossible, to see through the fog of grief to help anyone else. Your fog has become more dense.

If there are children, brothers or sisters, mothers or fathers, you must share this time with them, for their grief is great too. The caretaker in you usually kicks in during this time of suspension. The funeral sometimes becomes almost like a party. It is and should be a celebration of your loved one's life, as memories and laughter are shared. This is good, because the pain is held at bay for time periods. It is a cleansing for all.

Each person's grief is unique unto that individual, not only because they are unique, but also because their relationship with the individual was also. Again, the major difference in their space of grief and yours is they will go home to resume their life with spouses, children, friends, jobs. They still have their grief, but they have to, again, compartmentalize it according to responsibilities. Their lives immediately become busy and full, with 'normal.'

You are the one who is now 'half' of a whole, living in an empty house of memories. Depression is there for all of us. It is the dealing with it day by day that helps us to get through the period of fog. We know it will lift; we just don't know when. There is no timetable and no way to speed the natural order. The fog comes and goes and comes again.

Many times these other grieving persons, family and friends alike, reach a point where they feel they have adequately dealt with their grief and wonder why you have not. Sometimes they even verbalize this to you. I know it is hard, but try not to take offense.

REMEMBER THIS: They have not yet been in the place where you stand. They are well meaning; they just do not know. Remember my words: Do NOT judge; Do NOT compare.

If you could only sense how important you are to the lives of those you meet; how important you can be to the people you may never even dream of. There is something of yourself that you leave at every meeting with another person.

—— Fred Rogers

The World According to Mister Rogers

WHERE DO WE FIND GOD (AGAIN)?

I said this was not a religious book; however, I would be terribly remiss without this section because I do believe this book was God inspired and directed.

I find God in the early morning hours.

Years ago our priest (and best friend), Allen Cooke, suggested we 'take on' something, rather than giving up something for Lent. I began to get up an hour earlier (at that time in my life my daughters were still in school and there seemed to be no other time in my busy life) to read the Bible. Another Lent I 'tried' to write a note to someone everyday (this one took several Lents to fulfill).

You guessed it! This became a precious habit. It became my time with God. I would sit in the living room early in the morning, with coffee, read, and pray. After my husband died, I established a new routine. I had coffee in bed with God each morning. I still do this. My time with God has lengthened each morning, as we share readings from different books.

God has sustained me. He has often carried me. I cannot imagine going through 'the worst' without Him by my side. Perhaps you are not there yet. Perhaps you have not 'talked' with God in a long time (or ever). Perhaps you are angry with God. All of this is OK. All it takes to turn the corner is desire. Just listen. God is there.

Marlo Thomas wrote in her second book, *The Right Words at the Right Time*, of a young woman whose husband had died of cancer, leaving her alone with an eleven year old son. With a 'shakey' relationship with God, she picked out a synagogue in the Yellow Pages and went there and screamed and yelled at God for an hour, venting her anger. Afterwards she went to the Rabbi and told him what she had done and how guilty she felt. He smiled gently and said, "At least it's a relationship." Another story in her book was of a young Catholic woman whose faith and training had begun to unravel when she had gone off to college. Sitting alone in church, questioning if there is a God, a nun sat down beside her and listened to her turmoil. After her speel, the nun asked softly, " Do you believe in people, in their being born with good intentions?" The young woman replied, "I think so." The nun gave her these words, "Then you believe in God. That's good enough for now."

The point is – your anger is OK. "At least it's a relationship. That's good enough for now."

Jerry Sittser lost his wife, his daughter, and his mother in a tragic car accident. He was left to raise three young children, as well as rebuild his own life. He wrote in his book, *A Grace Disguised*, " My faith did not begin with the accident. Still, since then I have grown spiritually in new ways."

My husband and I grew together spiritually. I have had to learn to grow singularly. I have made new friends doing so, as well as deeper friendships with others. Try it. You won't be alone.

Learn to live one day at a time. By an act of your will, choose to start enjoying your life right now. Enjoy everything in your life.

—— Joel Osteen

What can "I" do?

For those of you who would ask, "So what can I do?" I would say – just be there. You, too, should not judge or compare.

I saved this reading from a *Day by Day*:

Our culture wants to push people through despair, depression, grief. "Get over it," we say (or think) when someone else's suffering makes us uncomfortable. But sometimes we are called to simply ***be*** *. . . to be with someone in the midst of anguish, without trying to solve the situation.*

Sometimes the hardest thing to do is simply to stand still, not to turn away, not to run away from another's passion or pain. Be there. Just be there.

Just be a friend. Realize the importance of friendship. Help someone else. I saved this quote a good friend sent:

Each friend represents a world in us, a world possibly not born until they arrive, and it is only by this meeting that a new world is born.

—— Anais Nir

God speaks to us in many ways . . . Listen to the Whispers

—— epl

JOY

Will I ever know joy again?

Listen to me and know what I say is true. Yes, joy does return. Just as I have said, one day you wake up and "know" you want to live; one day you will realize you have suddently experienced 'joy' in a happening or person. It is a turning point.

Just as we are creating a new life, in this new chapter, in this second chance of life, our joy will no doubt be different too. We must find this new joy ourselves – outside the realm of caregiving. As we learn to give care to ourselves, we have to listen carefully for a new awakening of joy – joy in the ordinary, i.e., growing a garden, cooking gourmet meals, painting, writing, returning to school, volunteering, helping someone else, helping ourselves . . . stepping out-of-our box.

Pamela Peeks uses 'joy' as a verb, asking her patients to pay attention to daily joys by saying, *"So – Have you joyed yourself today?"*

Begin to develop new rituals – just for you!

-Have a Tea Time – just for you

-Start a 'walking' group

-Plan mini trips with different people

-Start a book club

-Try a new recipe once a week (month)

-Go out to lunch/dinner with someone new
-Do something anonymously for someone else
-Be creative – step out-of-your box

"Joy" yourself today!

Giving anonymously is divine.

—— Alexandra Stoddard

A New Beginning

Linda Feinberg wrote, "I don't even know what's normal anymore." We all know the truth of that statement. We have to develop a new 'normal.' I am beginning my Third Life. I owe it to myself to make it the best life I can. I owe it to the memory of my husband to enhance the personal growth that we shared and to go beyond. This is a big year for me, and this book is my personal gift to myself. It has taken me awhile to get to this place, but that's OK too.

REMEMBER this quote that has been so hard for me:

> *We must be willing to get rid of the life we've planned,*
> *So as to have the life that is waiting for us.*
>
> —— Joseph Campbell

At a recent wedding of a nephew, the groom's father and my brother, Mike (a Baptist minister), prayed that they have "an interesting journey" together. I like that. Let's make this life, this second chance, an interesting journey too.

Cassandra King wrote in *Queen of Broken Hearts*, *"What have we learned about loss during our time together? Hopefully we've found that loss is always a journey of self-discovery. And now we know that the journey has not ended; It has just begun."*

Listen to the Whispers . . .

—— epl

AND SO . . .

I would like to express my sincere gratitude to all whose words I have borrowed to enhance my work, for in those words, I have found solace. I hope you do also. May we all help someone else.

In January of 2006, a friend gave me some statistics she had read. In a year, 700,000 become widows. Of those, 30,000 remarry.

REMEMBER THIS: That is only 2%. This is a strong argument for rebuilding ourselves as individuals.

For some years now, our church has compiled a pamphlet of meditations for Lent, written by lay volunteers and based on four Biblical verses for that day. During the last years of his life, my husband chose to participate with a Good Friday writing. He ended with this:

Today is the day that Jesus died for us; and, because of this, our own death is not an ending but a new beginning, not a day of sorrow but one of celebration, and not a day of remorse but one of thanksgiving. Thanks be to God!

His favorite Bible verse: *I can do all things through Christ who strengthens me.* Phil. 4:13

. . . .

The quotes I give in this book and at the end that I have shared with you have touched a part of me at some point in my life. They were given to me at times when I needed them.

REMEMBER THIS: Just because something speaks to me, it may not be speaking to you. That's OK. When I give a special book to a friend, I also say, if it doesn't speak to you now, lay it aside and pick it up at a later date. Time travels differently for all.

Listen to the Whispers . . .

—— epl

You make your own happiness.

—— Rudy Lane

Notes

It is with gratitude that I note the following writings that have traveled with me on my journey.

Dominique Browning
Around the House and In The Garden

Always . . . my Day by Day readings

Lisa Gardner
Gone (novel)

Margaret Whitmore Hickman
Healing After Loss (given to me by Adrienne Ford)
This book has been read three times in full and many times in highlight; it has been given to many others in need.

Roger Housden
Seven Sins For a Life Worth Living

Cassandra King
Queen of Broken Hearts (novel)

Charlotte King
A Letter to Friends

Caroline Myss
Invisible Acts of Power

Oprah
"O" Magazine

Joel Osteen
Your Best Life Now — Book and Journal
(given to me by Beth Jeffers)

Don Piper
90 Minutes in Heaven
(given by Beth Jeffers)

Nora Roberts

Black Rose (novel)

Divided in Death (novel)

Florence Scovel Shinn

The Wisdom of Florence Scovel Shinn

(recommended by Wendy Van Pelt Gautney)

Jerry Sittser

A Grace Disguised

(recommended by Jan Hardeman)

Marlo Thomas

The Right Words at the Right Time

(discovered on a visit to granddaughter, Whitney Jeffers, in Oxford, Mississippi)

C.S. Lewis

A Grief Observed

(recommended by Barbara Broach)

Joan Didion
The Year of Magical Thinking
(recommended by Barbara Broach)

Alexandra Stoddard
ALL 23 books
(especially — *Choosing Happiness*)
given by Paige and Robyn

Suffice it to say, these need listing; however, truth be known, and after the first three months, many, many books and authors could be listed. For those who truly enjoy reading, you will understand — books are friends, friends who bring healing.

Angels Unaware . . . Thank God for things that happen without reason.

— epl

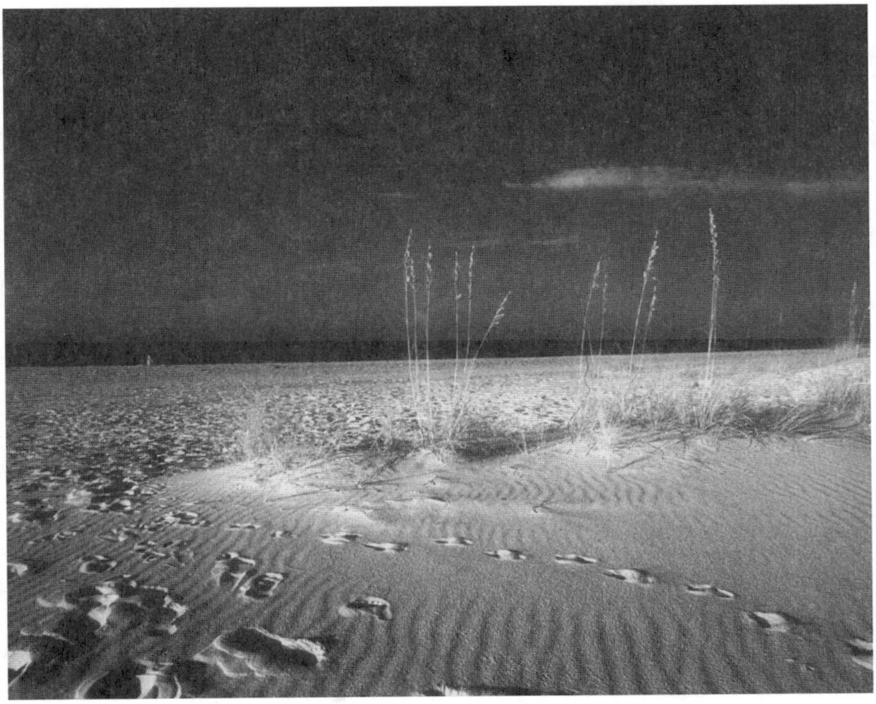

Footsteps in the Sand by Terry M. Purdy

Listen to the Whispers . . .